ADVANCE STATEMENTS ABOUT
MEDICAL TREATMENT

ADVANCE STATEMENTS ABOUT MEDICAL TREATMENT

CODE OF PRACTICE
with Explanatory Notes

Report of the
British Medical Association

Published by the BMJ Publishing Group
Tavistock Square, London WC1H 9JR
April 1995

First published in 1995

British Library Cataloguing in Publication Data
A catalogue record for this book is available from the British Library

ISBN 07279 09142

Printed in Great Britain by Derry & Sons Ltd. Nottingham

Membership of the Steering Group

Mr Derek Morgan, Chairman	Cardiff Law School; Member BMA Medical Ethics Committee
Ms June Andrews	Board Secretary, Royal College of Nursing, Scotland
Ms Alison Britton	Lawyer, Glasgow University Institute of Law & Ethics in Medicine
Ms Helen Caulfield	Legal Officer, Royal College of Nursing
Ms Veronica English	Senior Research Officer, BMA Ethics Department
Mr Chris Heginbotham	Chief Executive, Riverside Mental Health Trust
Professor Simon Lee	Law Department, Queens University, Belfast
Professor David London	Registrar, Royal College of Physicians
Mr Denzil Lush	Lawyer, Anstey, Sargent & Probert
Dr Stephen Luttrell	Geriatric Department, Whittington Hospital
Mr Indarjit Singh	Member, BMA Medical Ethics Committee
Ms Ann Sommerville	Advisor to the BMA on Medical Ethics
Dr Joseph Stoddart	Consultant in Anaesthesia & Intensive Therapy; Royal College of Anaesthetists
Dr Ben Sweeny	Chairman, Ethics Committee, Royal College of General Practitioners
Mr Jim Waits	Chief Executive, Worcester District Health Authority
Dr Michael Wilks	Member, BMA Medical Ethics Committee

Observers

Dr Elaine Gadd	Department of Health
Ms Claire Johnston	English Law Commission
Ms Penny Letts	English Law Society
Mr David Nichols	Scottish Law Commission

Written by	Ms Ann Sommerville
Contributor	Professor Andrew Grubb
Editor	Mr Derek Morgan
Editorial Secretary	Ms Gillian Romano
Project Manager	Miss Rosemary Weston

Contents

PART I

Background

1 Introduction

This guidance is a response to the House of Lords Select Committee on Medical Ethics, which in 1994 called for a Code of Practice on advance directives for health professionals. A multi-professional group under the aegis of the British Medical Association and medical and nursing Royal Colleges undertook the task of drafting it. Oral and written evidence was received from a wide range of individuals and groups. We wish to thank them for their help.

The Code takes a broad and essentially practical approach. It considers a range of advance statements, rather than limiting itself to those which have "directive" force. It advises that there are both benefits and dangers to making treatment decisions in advance. Health professionals and patients should be aware of both. Nevertheless, carefully discussed advance statements have an important place in the development of a genuinely more balanced partnership between patients and health professionals. Inevitably, the concept of shared decision-making implies a renegotiation of the traditional scope of clinical discretion in favour of accommodating patients' views. This is part of a growing trend of people taking greater personal responsibility for their health. It is to be welcomed.

Special importance attaches to a person's desire to make the manner of their dying consistent with the pattern of their life.

1

But sensitive and compassionate management of death is only one aspect of a longer dialogue about choice which should occur between those giving and those needing health care. The Code does not restrict advance statements to discussions about death but recognises their potential value in other situations where people wish to influence what happens to them after the onset of mental incapacity. Nevertheless, advance statements appear to have only limited value in relation to the treatment of recurrent episodic mental illness. This is a unique area in which patients are unable to refuse the compulsory detention and treatment for mental disorder authorised by mental health legislation, although notice of their preferred treatment options may be helpful.

We endorse the recommendation of the Select Committee that health professionals should have training appropriate to their ethical responsibilities. Training must include the skills of sensitive communication and receptivity. Sensitive, continuing dialogue is given high priority, for example, in the palliative care setting which provides some effective models of oral advance statements.

1.1 This Code reflects good clinical practice in encouraging dialogue about individuals' wishes concerning their future treatment. It does not address euthanasia, assisted suicide or methods for allocating health service resources. These are entirely separate from advance statements.

1.2 At all stages of life, timely discussion of treatment options is an important part of the duty of care owed by health professionals to those who consult them. Recognising and respecting the individual patient's values and preferences are fundamental aspects of good practice.

The Code seeks to divorce "advance directives" from practices of euthanasia and assisted suicide and places statements and directives within an accepted framework of discussion and communication.

2 Definitions

2.1 *Advance statements:* People who understand the implications of their choices can state in advance how they wish to be treated if they suffer loss of mental capacity. Just as adults must be consulted about treatment options, young people under the age of majority (age 18) are entitled to have their views taken into account. An advance statement (sometimes known as a living will) can be of various types (see also figure 1):

- a requesting statement reflecting an individual's aspirations and preferences. This can help health professionals identify how the person would like to be treated without binding them to that course of action, if it conflicts with professional judgement.

- a statement of the general beliefs and aspects of life which an individual values. This provides a summary of individual responses to a list of questions about a person's past and present wishes and future desires. It makes no specific request or refusal but attempts to give a biographical portrait of the individual as an aid to deciding what he or she would want.

- a statement which names another person who should be consulted at the time a decision has to be made. The views expressed by that named person should reflect what the patient would want. This can supplement and clarify the intended scope of a written statement but the named person's views are presently not legally binding in England & Wales. In Scotland, the powers of a tutor dative may cover such eventualities.

- a clear instruction refusing some or all medical procedures (advance directive). Made by a competent adult, this does, in certain circumstances, have legal force.

- a statement which, rather than refusing any particular treatment, specifies a degree of irreversible deterioration (such as a diagnosis of persistent vegetative state) after

which no life sustaining treatment should be given. For adults, this again can have legal force.

- **a combination of the above, including requests, refusals and the nomination of a representative. Those sections expressing clear refusal may have legal force in the case of adult patients.**

An advance statement can be a written document, a witnessed oral statement, a signed printed card, a smart card or a note of a discussion recorded in the patient's file. Only a clear refusal of particular treatment by an adult has potential legal force. Clear general statements of preferences should be respected if appropriate but are not legally binding. Any advance statement (whether a consent or refusal, written or oral) is superseded by a clear and competent contemporaneous decision by the

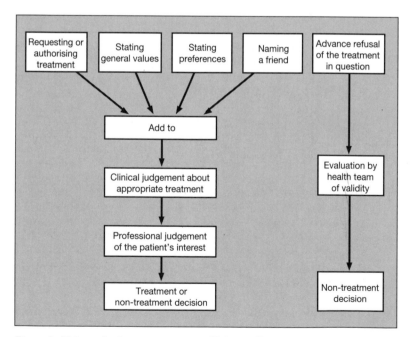

Figure 1. ***Types of advance statement (living will)***

individual concerned. In the case of young people under the age of majority (age 18), advance statements should be taken into account and accommodated if possible but can be overruled by a court or a person with parental responsibility.

Medical treatment decisions are seldom choices made once for all time but involve a series of steps as a patient's clinical condition changes and his or her understanding of the real and potential implications develops. Profoundly life-affecting treatment decisions are often made against a background of uncertainty, since medicine itself is uncertain and because new techniques are constantly evolving. The progress or remission of a disease can be affected by physiological or psychological factors unique to the individual. Each stage of treatment involves discussion between patients and health professionals. Loss of mental capacity robs people of the opportunity to participate in the dialogue or to re-assess their options. Advance statements are an imperfect substitute, but for some they are the only means of expressing their wishes about what they want to happen.

2.2 *Advance directives* (refusals): Competent, informed adults have an established legal right to refuse medical procedures in advance. An unambiguous and informed advance refusal is as valid as a contemporaneous decision. Health professionals are bound to comply when the refusal specifically addresses the situation which has arisen. Refusal is a serious matter, ideally to be considered in discussion with health professionals.

Since no-one can demand that medical treatment be given, statements purporting to "direct" or instruct health professionals are necessarily refusals. Although a clear refusal is potentially legally binding, a refusal seriously likely to affect other people adversely (such as exposing them to the risk of harm) may be invalidated. This includes a refusal of basic care measures.

Competent adults have an established legal right to reject medical advice, assessment or treatment, except in cases where this harms others or conflicts with legislation (see section 4).

What can be refused contemporaneously can also be refused in advance. All advance decisions carry some risk of error in evaluating possible future events and feelings. The legally binding nature of a competent advance refusal may increase the gravity of the risk. When people decide to take on these risks, it is important that health professionals provide factual information to help them (see section 6). Young people under the age of majority cannot make legally binding treatment refusals although their wishes should be taken into consideration.

2.3 *Care*: **Basic care means those procedures essential to keep an individual comfortable. The administration of medication or the performance of any procedure which is <u>solely or primarily</u> designed to provide comfort to the patient or alleviate that person's pain, symptoms or distress are facets of basic care. In each case, health professionals must continually assess the scope of measures essential for the patient's comfort. Although the law on this matter is not clear, this Code provides that as a matter of public policy, people should not be able to refuse basic care in advance or instruct others to refuse it on their behalf (see also section 5).**

The adult patient's right to refuse medical interventions is well recognised by the common law. There are no clearly defined limits as to the sort of care or treatment which an informed, competent adult can refuse. Statutory powers under public health and mental health legislation, however, recognise a public interest in limiting in exceptional cases an individual's freedom to refuse medical examination and hospitalisation. These laws are based on the presumption that people cannot exercise their freedom in a manner which puts others at risk of harm. The Code reflects the view that a certain minimal level of intervention ("basic care") should be given notwithstanding a patient's refusal, since failure to do so exposes nurses, doctors and possibly other patients to unacceptable harms or burdens.

Defining "basic care" is problematic. A definition too tightly drawn may lead to unintentional omissions; whereas a definition which is too wide gives rise to uncertainty. In the face of an apparently valid refusal of all interventions, the Code recommends that only those measures *essential* for patient comfort can be given. These will require constant reappraisal in each individual case and attention must be paid to the individual's verbal and non-verbal indications of his or her comfort needs. It is generally accepted that basic care includes warmth, shelter, pain relief, management of distressing symptoms, such as breathlessness and vomiting, and hygiene measures, such as management of incontinence. Recognising that near the end of life, patients seldom want nutrition or hydration, basic care would nevertheless include measures such as moistening a patient's mouth as necessary for comfort.

This is a controversial area where lawyers and courts may differ. The Code advises that since the comfort of the mentally incapacitated person is the prime criterion, appropriate food or drink should be made available for (but not forced upon) those who manifest a clear desire for it. The implication of this recommendation is that an advance refusal of oral feeding can be withdrawn by a person who retains sufficient mental capacity to indicate a desire for it. Nutrition and hydration should not be given to a person who indicates opposition. Invasive measures such as tube feeding should not be instituted contrary to a clear advance refusal.

In cases of disagreement or the need for greater clarity on the issue of refusal of basic care in an individual case, application should be made to the courts for clarification.

2.4 *Capacity:* indicates an ability to understand the implications of the particular decision which the individual purports to make. The High Court has held that a person has capacity if he or she can understand and retain the information relevant to the decision in question, can believe that information and can weigh that information in the balance to arrive at a choice[1]. (For assessment of capacity, see section 8).

---

1   Re C *(Adult: Refusal of Medical Treatment)* [1994] 1 WLR 290

"Capacity" is a legal term. Capacity and competence are used interchangeably in this document. People who lack the ability to understand the ramifications of financial decisions, for example, may well understand the implications of medical treatment. A distinction is drawn between an ability to understand and the fact of having actually understood. People who possess the ability may make an invalid decision if it has not been explained in a manner they can be said to have understood. Although they may understand and weigh the implications, young people under the age of majority do not have the same rights at law as an adult (see section 4).

PART II

Making Treatment Choices

3 Making Treatment Choices

3.1 Adults can refuse clinical procedures contemporaneously or in advance of deteriorating mental capacity. Although no parallel right to insist upon a specific procedure or to order one of various treatment options is recognised in law, dialogue with patients about the choices facing them is an essential part of ethical health-care. Patients may properly expect to be provided with the details they need in an accessible form to allow them to make informed choices.

Statements expressing requests or preferences are not legally binding but should be respected and complied with if appropriate. Patients may prefer not to make a legalistic document but to talk to a doctor or nurse about their wishes and have these reflected in their notes. In such cases, patients should be encouraged to check the notes made about them to ensure they agree with what is written.

3.2 Discussion of options should be responsive to a patient's actual anxieties rather than trying to shape the patient's wishes to a preconceived standard format.

Patients may feel it is less threatening to talk about future options in a GP or outpatient setting. Continuous discussion, noted in the patient record, is a pattern which has developed in British palliative care services. Although we recognise there may be value in developing a standard format for advance statements, in practice this would be likely to undervalue those alternative methods for expressing preferences, including an oral statement.

3.3 Many personal, non-clinical issues influence how competent people reach decisions. When decisions are made on behalf of people who cannot choose for themselves, their previously expressed wishes and values should be taken into account.

It is principally for the individual to decide what is right for him or herself. The best outcome from a clinical perspective, although an important part of the evaluation, is seldom the sole consideration for an individual. Health professionals have legal and ethical obligations to act in the best interests of those for whom they have undertaken a duty of care. Judgement of what constitutes an individual's best interests rests upon the ascertainable past and present wishes and feelings of the individual as well as clinical factors.

3.4 An advance directive is not restricted to care in hospital. It may also cover care at home, in a nursing home or in a hospice.

There may be misapprehensions that advance directives (refusals), which can have legal force, only apply in certain locations or if counter-signed by a doctor as witness. No such requirements are recognised at common law.

4 The Legal Position

4.1 Common law establishes that an informed refusal of treatment made in advance by an adult who understands the implications of that decision has the same legal power as a contemporaneous refusal. In order to be legally binding, the individual must have envisaged the

type of situation which has subsequently arisen. In all circumstances, a contemporaneous decision by a competent individual overrides previously expressed statements by that person.

4.1.1 Consent and treatment refusal

A conscious, mentally competent adult cannot be given treatment without his or her valid consent. Consent may not be valid if insufficient relevant information is given. It is illegal and unethical to treat an adult who is capable of understanding and willing to know, unless the nature of the procedure, its purpose and implications have been explained and that person's agreement obtained.

The right to refuse screening, diagnostic procedures or treatment can be for reasons which are "rational, irrational or for no reason".[2] The Court of Appeal held in 1992 that an adult is entitled to refuse treatment, irrespective of the wisdom of that decision.[3] For the refusal to be valid, however, health professionals must be satisfied that the patient's capacity at the time of deciding was not affected by illness, medication, false information or pressure from other people (see section 8 for assessing mental capacity). Discussing the legal duties of health professionals in relation to a patient's refusal of treatment Lord Donaldson stated that:

"Doctors faced with a refusal of consent have to give very careful and detailed consideration to the patient's capacity to decide at the time when the decision was made. It may not be the simple case of the patient having no capacity because, for example, at that time he had hallucinations. It may be the more difficult case of reduced capacity at the time when his decision was made. What matters is that the doctors should consider whether at that time he had capacity which was

---

2   per Lord Templeton in *Sidaway v Board of Governors of the Bethlem Royal Hospital and Maudsley Hospital* [1985] AC 871

3   *Re T (Adult: Refusal of Treatment)* [1993] Fam 95.

commensurate with the gravity of the decision which he purported to make. The more serious the decision, the greater the capacity required. If the patient had the requisite capacity, they are bound by his decision. If not, they are free to treat him in what they believe to be his best interests".[4]

4.1.2   Advance consent

Some advance statements provide not only for refusal of treatment but for the option of asking "to be kept alive for as long as reasonably possible using whatever forms of treatment are available". To the extent that they demand the continuation of futile treatment or treatment which the health care team can no longer justify as serving the patient's best interests, they have no legal force. They may also permit personal requests such as preservation of life until a particular nominated person can be called to the bedside to say goodbye. One of the important points about this type of statement is that it shows that advance decision-making concerns a *right to choose* rather than a *right to die*.

4.1.3   Advance refusal

Adults who are capable of making current medical decisions for themselves can, if properly informed of the implications and consequences, also refuse in advance medical treatment which might be necessary when their capacity will be impaired. In the *Bland case*,[5] Lord Goff of Chieveley said "it has been held that a patient of sound mind may, if properly informed, require that life support should be discontinued. The same principle applies where the patient's refusal to give his consent has been expressed at an earlier date, before he became unconscious or otherwise incapable of communicating it".

The patient must have possessed insight into the implications of refusing treatment at the time of making the advance refusal

---

4   Lord Donaldson in *Re T (Adult: Refusal of Treatment)* [1993] Fam 95

5   *Airedale NHS Trust v Bland* [1993] AC 789.

in order for it to be valid. It is irrelevant whether the refusal is contrary to the views of most other people or whether the person lacks insight into other aspects of life as long as he or she is able to decide on the one matter in question. When a Broadmoor patient refused amputation of his gangrenous foot, the High Court held this to be a valid refusal currently and for the future, despite the fact that the man held demonstrably erroneous views on other matters.[6]

4.2 **Young people under the age of majority do not have the same rights at law as adults. It is good practice, however, for children and young people to be kept as fully informed as possible about their care and treatment. The Children Act 1989 emphasises that the views of minors should be sought and taken into account in matters which touch on their welfare. Where appropriate, they should be encouraged to take decisions jointly with those with whom they have a close relationship, especially parents.**

Competent patients of any age should feel confident that their views count and are respected. Children and young people do not have the same legal rights as adults and should be informed that, although efforts will be made to meet their wishes, in cases of disagreement about measures conducive to their welfare their own views will not necessarily be determinative. Discussion with young people should be structured so as to help them identify their own wants and needs but they should also be encouraged to take decisions jointly with those with whom they have a close relationship, especially parents.

4.3 **Advance statements are not covered by legislation. In cases of conflict with other legal provisions, advance statements are superseded by existing statute. The terms of the Mental Health Acts take precedence and must prevail regarding treatment for mental disorder.**

---

6   *Re C (Adult: Refusal of Medical Treatment)* [1994] 1 WLR 290

A compulsorily detained adult can make a legally binding advance refusal of treatment _not_ covered by the mental health legislation. Where appropriate, patients' preferences should be included in treatment plans for both informal and detained patients.

There is no statute on advance statements although common law recognises the legal force of advance directives (refusals of treatment). Nevertheless even clear and specific advance directives (refusals) are superseded by existing Acts of Parliament. Conflict might arise between an advance directive, which would otherwise be legally binding, and the legal authority to give treatment under the Mental Health Acts. The provisions of the Mental Health Act 1983, Mental Health (Scotland) Act 1984, and the Mental Health (Northern Ireland) Order 1986 authorise the assessment of individuals, their admission to hospital or to guardianship and if necessary medical treatment or care without their consent. A patient may be compulsorily admitted to hospital under the Act where it is necessary:

in the interests of his or her own health; or

in the interests of his or her own safety; or

for the protection of other people.[7]

Any provisions of advance directives refusing treatment of mental illness are rendered invalid in circumstances where the patient is legally detained for treatment.

Treatment under the Mental Health Act 1983 in England and Wales is covered by guidance given in the Code of Practice,[8] chapter 15 of which discusses the principles of patient consent in the context of treatment for mental disorder. It emphasises the

---

7   See para 2.6 of Mental Health Act Code of Practice, HMSO, August 1993 (England and Wales). Similar Codes of Practice have also been issued for Scotland (Mental Health Act: Code of Practice (Scotland)) and for Northern Ireland (Code of Practice for Mental Health Orders (N. Ireland)).

8   _supra_

importance of treatment plans for both informal and detained patients, including advice about the desirability, wherever possible, of discussing the whole plan with the patient. Patients' advance statements or preferences regarding treatment options should also be included in the plan and in the discussion of immediate and long-term goals. Any part of an advance statement or directive (refusal) which refers to medical treatment outside the scope of the mental health legislation requires careful consideration.

5 Public Policy

5.1 Advance statements refusing basic care and maintenance of an incompetent person's comfort should not, as a matter of public policy, be binding on care providers. Although the law on this matter is not free from doubt, this Code provides that people should not be able to refuse basic care in advance or instruct others to refuse it on their behalf.

Personal autonomy, although important, cannot always be an overriding ethical principle. In most situations, the individual's right to refuse treatment outweighs any competing interests, including the wishes of other people. In exceptional circumstances, the individual's choice has unacceptable consequences, such as potentially serious harm for others which is sufficient to outweigh the patient's right of refusal. Others may be harmed if refusal of basic care leads, for example, to the spread of infection.

Caring for a person whose pain or symptoms are not sufficiently relieved as a result of an advance refusal may impose an intolerable burden on those around them, and abandonment of an incapacitated person is unacceptable.

Our view, that individuals cannot validly refuse basic care, does not necessarily imply that health professionals are obliged to provide every facet of basic care. They should, rather, provide that which is reasonable in the circumstances. Some patients are prepared to tolerate a degree of discomfort and reduced medication, for example, in order to remain sufficiently alert to enjoy the company of visitors. Particularly in a palliative care setting, medical and nursing procedures are continually adjusted to suit the patient's requirements without infringing upon those of other patients or carers.

5.2 In the absence of an advance statement by a person who is now incapable of deciding, health professionals have a duty to act in that person's best interests.

5.3 Relatives' views may help in clarifying a patient's wishes but relatives' opinions cannot overrule those of the patient or supplant health professionals' duty to assess the patient's best interest.

The assessment of a person's best interests includes consideration of what he or she would have wanted, if that can be discerned from people close to the patient or from previous remarks recorded in the patient's notes (see also section 10 on implementation).

PART III

Drafting

6   Making an Advance Statement

6.1   Although oral statements are equally valid if supported by appropriate evidence, there are advantages to recording one's general views and firm decisions in writing. Advance statements should be understood as an aid to, rather than a substitute for, open dialogue between patients and health professionals.

Opportunistic or casual remarks by a healthy person reflecting distaste for life-prolonging treatment in the hypothetical event of incapacity are unlikely to meet the evidential requirements ·necessary to indicate an informed and considered decision. A general expression of views cannot be accorded the same weight as a firm decision. If representative of consistently manifested values, however, oral remarks contribute to the evaluation of the patient's interests. If witnessed and made by an informed individual, they could carry legal weight.

Many patients only lose capacity shortly before death. If suffering from illness requiring long-term in-patient or out-patient care, they have opportunities for discussion with the health-care team over a long period. They may feel their wishes are sufficiently well known or reflected in the notes so that there is no need to write them down. In hospice or specialist palliative care settings, this form of oral advance statement or directive (refusal) is common practice and appears to be respected.

In other situations, there is a risk that written advance statements might reduce rather than enhance the opportunities for discussion since inhibitions about raising the matter with health professionals lead some people to draft them in isolation. Individuals making an advance statement have to cope with difficult questions of their own mortality and loss of mental abilities as well as preparing for the fact that others may have to make crucial decisions of life and death for them. In such a situation, the patient will need counselling.

6.2 Written statements should use clear and unambiguous language. They should be signed by the individual and a witness. Model forms are available but clear statements in any format command respect.

There are no specific legal requirements concerning the format of the statement. The minimum requirements for the statement to be legally valid concern only the individual's competence, awareness of the implications of the decision and the relevance of the decision to the circumstances which arise (see section 4).

It is clear that some people have a false impression that a written, witnessed statement carries more weight than their contemporaneous oral consent or refusal and so make statements for the wrong reasons. Health professionals must be aware of this and make all reasonable efforts to prevent such misunderstanding.

Health professionals can give advice that will lead to a well balanced declaration and they should be aware that their opinions and attitudes are likely to be influential even if they personally do not see the importance of writing an advance statement. They should record the patient's wishes about treatment and non-treatment in their own notes.

6.3 Patients have a legitimate expectation of being provided with information in an accessible form to allow them to make informed choices. Health professionals should ensure that the foreseeable options and implications are adequately explained, admit to uncertainty when this is the case and make reasonable efforts to discover if there is more specialised information available to pass on to the patient. An open attitude on the part of health professionals and a willingness to discuss the advantages and disadvantages of certain options can do much to establish trust and mutual understanding.

Foreseeable deterioration of mental faculties should be raised sensitively so that people can plan ahead without being pushed into committing themselves to a particular course. Any diagnosis of a life-threatening illness or deteriorating mental capacity must be backed by support and information so that patients can understand how their previous expectations for the future will be affected. The giving and receiving of bad news is likely to mark a new stage in the relationship between the patient and those providing health care. The existence of opportunities and receptiveness to discussion will affect how both sides experience the patient's illness. Insensitivity or lack of communication impacts on both. Good communication is not an optional extra service but an essential part of health care. It is important that health professionals have access to training in effective communication skills, and that there is a significant take-up of these opportunities.

GP practices may establish counselling and support sessions for people with conditions such as Alzheimer's Disease. Funding may come from the GP's Health Promotion Budget. Some surgeries and hospitals make available leaflets to help people consider treatment options in advance. People should be encouraged to take time to consider the issues carefully and ask questions. Routine consultation with the GP or practice nurse can provide such opportunities. Continuing specialist consultations, such as pain management clinics, also allow options to be discussed over a period of time.

6.4 Admittance to hospital, with its associated anxieties, is not generally a good time to raise the subject of anticipatory choice. Exceptions arise when the impetus for discussion comes from the patient or when sensitive advance discussion of cardiopulmonary resuscitation would be appropriate.

Admittance to hospital for treatment is stressful. Nevertheless, discussion of treatment options will sometimes arise then, either at the patient's initiation or because the patient's views need to be sought about cardiopulmonary resuscitation (CPR). Discussion of resuscitation with all patients is inappropriate. The benefit and the patient's views may be beyond doubt, or there may be no expectation of CPR providing medical benefit. Sensitive exploration of the patient's wishes about CPR should be undertaken with patients who are at risk of cardiac or respiratory failure or who have a terminal illness. Ideally this should be done by the consultant. The views of the patient, where these can be ascertained, should be documented in the patient's records.

6.5 Advance statements should not be made under pressure. Professionals consulted at the drafting stage should take reasonable steps to ensure patients' decisions are not made under duress. Statements may evolve in stages over a period of time and discussion. It is inadvisable to conclude refusals or complicated statements in one discussion without further review. Patients should be reminded about the desirability of reviewing their statement on a regular basis, although a statement made long in advance is not automatically invalidated.

Time and support are required to come to terms with the full implications of bad news. Some people make clear that they do not want to know or else accept the knowledge in progressive stages. After considering the options, some patients will prefer decisions to be made for them by health professionals or other people they trust.

Health professionals and lawyers are often consulted at the time of drafting an advance statement. If in the course of discussing the statement they suspect there may be duress, they should take steps to counter it. This might, for example, take the form of arranging independent counselling for the patient.

Statements made long in advance of incapacity are not invalid but a regularly reviewed document is more likely to be applicable to the circumstances. Views change over time and, as the House of Lords Select Committee noted, "disabled individuals are commonly more satisfied with their life than able-bodied people would expect to be with the same disability. The healthy do not choose in the same way as the sick".[9] A new stage in a patient's illness may be an appropriate time to review earlier stated wishes. Computerised annual recall facilities may be a way for GPs to remind patients to review their advance statements.

6.6 Patients should be advised to avoid rushing into specifying future treatment when they have only recently received a prognosis or when they may be unduly influenced by others or depressed.

6.7 Hospital managers and GP practice managers need to consider how to respond to the increasing desire by patients to plan ahead on the basis of accurate health information and advice.

There is no ideal moment to make an advance statement but there are clearly times which should be avoided. Health professionals providing information about prognosis or treatment options should advise patients of the risks of a premature or ill-considered decision.

Managers need to consider the provision of appropriately skilled staff, with time to discuss treatment implications. Giving bad news and helping patients make decisions on the basis of it is not a matter to be finalised on one occasion and adequate opportunities for discussion will need to be built into the

---

9   Report from the Select Committee on Medical Ethics, HMSO, 1994, Vol 1, p.41

health-care budget. Some hospitals retain specialised counsellors who provide information and support for in-patients and out-patients. With home visits they also have opportunities to discuss the options with other people who the patient wants to involve. Hospice outreach services and community nurses may also become involved in carrying out such a role. General practices and hospital policy makers will need to consider how to respond to patient demand for this type of service.

6.8 When responding to a request for assistance with advance statements, there are fundamental issues health professionals should consider:

- **Does the patient have sufficient knowledge of the medical condition and possible treatment options if there is a known illness?**

- **Is the patient mentally competent?**

- **Is it clear that the patient is reflecting his or her own views and is not being pressured by other people?**

Patients may have an unrealistic view of what medical science can or cannot do for them. Media reports sometimes result in an emotional declaration being written by people in a panic. There is a risk that such statements may take on a life of their own at a crucial moment without the writer having really foreseen the consequences. Impulsively written texts could be dangerous for the patient and confusing for the health team. Health professionals should attempt to give as much relevant factual information as possible in a form which the patient can assimilate. Often it will be difficult to avoid euphemisms and to give patients a clear view of the likely progression of the disease without also alarming or depressing them.

There are various opportunities for health professionals working in the community to discuss anticipatory decisions, such as when a person joins a GP practice or at times when regular health checks allow time for discussion with the doctor or practice nurse.

6.9 There are advantages and disadvantages to making antici-patory decisions. Advance refusals are likely to be legally binding. Health professionals should try to ensure that patients are aware of drawbacks as well as advantages.

People are influenced by the type of advice and information they receive and how the options are portrayed to them. They need accurate information about the potential advantages and disadvantages of deciding in advance. Advance statements can have psychological and other benefits. Initiating discussion may clarify choices and enhance trust. Recording decisions gives a sense of control and peace of mind. Anecdotal reports recount cases of statements stored away by people who apparently made no effort to communicate their wishes; the discussion and drafting exercise apparently being sufficient. Statements can guide health professionals in difficult cases and remove the burden on people close to the patient.

The disadvantages include the risks of pressure or other forms of abuse and the impossibility of predicting how one might adapt to disabilities. Misdiagnosis might occur and unforeseen treatments may be developed. People might forget to amend the statement if their views change. Badly drafted statements can mislead or cause confusion and result in patients being treated differently than they intended or not treated at all.

7 Contents of Advance Statements

7.1 Advance statements may list the individual's values as a basis for others to reach appropriate decisions. They may request all medically reasonable efforts be made to prolong life or express preferences between treat-ment options.

Advance statements can cover a range of matters, including both general views and specific decisions. Authorising statements (advance consent), although legally unenforceable, assist health professionals to accommodate decisions which are so personal that only the individual concerned could make them. A key concern for many people is to be able to say where they would like to be cared for and where they wish to die or who they want called to their bedside.

It is sometimes thought that clear and explicit advance refusals will most likely apply to futile treatments. Good professional practice should, in any event, ensure that these are not administered, and the courts have made clear that health professionals cannot be required to give treatment contrary to clinical judgement. Statements of advance consent are thus often seen as of more use and advance statements of views and preferences may be particularly helpful in non-emergency situations in determining what is in the patient's best interests.

7.2 Advance directives are specific refusals of treatment and can be legally binding (see section 4).

7.3 Adults cannot authorise or refuse in advance, procedures which they could not authorise or refuse contemporaneously. They cannot authorise unlawful procedures or insist upon futile or inappropriate treatment.

As a matter of public policy, we have also stated that people should not be able to require withdrawal of basic care and comfort measures (see section 5).

7.4 Women of child bearing age should be advised to consider the possibility of their advance statement or directive being invoked at a time when they are pregnant. A waiver covering pregnancy might be written into the statement.

7.5 If a patient is detained under the Mental Health Act, drugs with potentially damaging side effects may sometimes have to be prescribed without prior discussion with the patient. When the patient regains insight, advance statements about preferences between equally viable options for future treatment can be discussed and reflected in subsequent treatment plans.

Professionals providing mental health care have responsibilities for mentally disordered patients who may suffer recurrent psychotic episodes. If the patient has to be detained under the Mental Health Act, in some circumstances neuroleptics and other drugs (which may sometimes cause damaging side effects) may have to be prescribed without prior discussion with the patient. Once the patient recovers from a psychotic episode, health professionals have a key role in assisting the patient to evaluate and reconcile the advantages and disadvantages of the treatment and make decisions about future management accordingly. Anticipatory statements authorising treatment or expressing preferences between equally viable treatments can be discussed at times when the patient retains insight about the condition and these should be reflected in subsequent treatment plans. If, however, a patient is detained for compulsory treatment under Mental Health legislation, any advance refusal of treatment by the patient could be overruled (see section 4).

8   Assessing Mental Capacity

8.1   Opportunities for assessing mental capacity arise at two points. First, an individual must have enough under-standing of the implications in order to make a valid advance statement. Secondly, that statement will then speak for the patient at the point where he or she is considered to have insufficient understanding to make the particular decision in question.

Only when a person has or has had sufficient understanding and awareness to make a decision can significance attach to it. Capacity must always be assessed in relation to the decision in question. Health professionals are sometimes asked to make retrospective judgements about a patient's capacity. The BMA and the Law Society are producing detailed guidance for doctors and lawyers on this and other aspects of assessing capacity. A medical opinion about an individual's legal capacity may be open to challenge either by the person concerned or by another interested party.

8.2 When consulted by someone who wishes to draft an advance statement, health professionals should consider whether there are any reasons to doubt the patient's capacity to make the decisions in question. Capacity is assumed unless evidence suggests the contrary. The signature of a health professional as a witness may well imply that assessment of capacity has taken place.

The assessment of adult patients' capacities to make decisions about their own medical treatment is a matter for professional judgement guided by current practice and subject to legal requirements. Under normal circumstances, it is the personal responsibility of any health professional proposing to examine or to treat a patient to judge whether the patient has the capacity to give a valid consent. Similarly, if consulted to witness or assist in the drafting of an advance statement, health professionals should consider whether there are grounds for doubting the person's capacity and, if in doubt, seek a further opinion.

8.3 The High Court has held that a person has capacity if he or she can understand and retain the information relevant to the decision in question, can believe that information and can assess it in arriving at a choice.[10]

In order for an advance directive to be valid a patient must, at the time the statement was made, have had the capacity to understand and weigh the implications and consequences of that choice. The level of understanding required to make decisions must be commensurate with the gravity of the decision being made.

8.4 To demonstrate capacity individuals should be able to:

- **understand in broad terms and simple language what the medical treatment is, its purpose and nature and why it is or will be proposed for them;**

---

10   *Re C (Adult: Refusal of Medical Treatment)* [1994] 1WLR 290

- **understand its principal benefits, risks and alternatives;**

- **understand in broad terms what will be the consequences of not receiving the proposed treatment;**

- **make a free choice (ie free from undue pressure);**

- **retain the information long enough to make an effective decision.**

It must be remembered that:

— there is a presumption of capacity until the contrary is demonstrated;

— any assessment of an individual's capacity has to be made in relation to a particular treatment proposal;

— capacity in an individual with a mental disorder can be variable over time and so health professionals should attempt to identify the time and manner most helpful to the patient when they might discuss the matter;

— capacity may be temporarily impaired due to toxic conditions or extreme illness;

— all assessments of an individual's capacity should be fully recorded in the patient's medical, nursing and other appropriate notes.

9   Storage of Advance Statements

9.1 Storage of an advance statement and notification of its existence are primarily the responsibility of the individual. A copy of any written advance statement should be given to a person's General Practitioner. People close to the patient should be made aware of the existence of an advance statement and be told where it is.

Some individuals carry a card, bracelet or other measure indicating the existence of an advance statement and where it is kept.

9.2 For chronically ill patients, who are treated by a specialist team over a prolonged period, a copy of the advance statement should be in all relevant hospital files and the GP record.

Once an advance statement has been made, it should be readily accessible when the need arises. It is the responsibility of the individual to ensure that his or her statement is available. General statements, made by healthy individuals, are best lodged with their General Practitioner. This will allow the GP to provide the information to other health professionals on referral or, in emergency situations, to provide the information on request. For chronically ill patients, who are treated by a specialist team over a prolonged period, a copy of the advance statement should be in both relevant hospital files and the GP record.

PART IV

Implementation

10 General Implementation

10.1 If health professionals know or have reasonable grounds to believe that an advance statement exists and time permits, they should make further enquiries. This could be by looking in relevant hospital notes, or contacting the General Practitioner, or contacting people close to the patient.

Health professionals, once alerted to the existence of a relevant statement, should make reasonable efforts to find it. In an emergency where treatment delay might be fatal, clinical judgement must be exercised in deciding whether to follow the statement. When time permits, efforts must also be made to check the validity of any document presented. Basic verification includes checking that a written statement actually belongs to the patient who has been admitted, is dated, signed, preferably is witnessed and that there is no evidence to show it has been revoked.

10.2 Emergency treatment should not normally be delayed in order to look for an advance statement or refusal if there is no clear indication that one exists (see also figure 2).

The principle of necessity allows health professionals to provide treatment (or to restrain medically or physically a person who may commit harm) without consent. The necessity justification applies mainly to emergency situations. Although the legal ground upon which such a justification is based is one of necessity, the language of consent may also be used. Consent in certain circumstances is 'implied' or 'presumed' or can be assumed will be obtained in the future.

If a person is now incapacitated but is known to have objections to all or some treatment, health professionals may not be justified in proceeding, even in an emergency. They will need to consider the available evidence about the patient's views and how convincing it seems. A written, witnessed statement should be viewed as convincing unless contradictory evidence of a retraction is available. Previous oral statements refusing treatment may be valid but also require evaluation of the evidence. In the absence of evidence of refusal, treatment which is in the interests of that individual can be given.

If the incapacity is temporary because of anaesthetic, sedation, intoxication or temporary unconsciousness, health professionals should not proceed beyond what is essential to preserve the person's life or prevent deterioration in health. In other words, treatments which are 'necessary', in that it would generally be agreed to be unreasonable to postpone them, are to be distinguished from those which are merely convenient. Treatment which could reasonably be postponed until the patient regains competency should not be given.

10.3 In England, Wales and Northern Ireland, no-one is legally empowered to consent or refuse on behalf of an adult who lacks capacity to make the particular treatment decision.

10.4 In Scotland, some treatment decisions may be taken by a tutor dative.

The views of people close to the patient can be helpful in identifying what he or she would want. Long-stay patients may also have discussed their wishes with nurses and other staff.

When an adult lacks mental capacity to make or communicate the particular treatment decision, no other person is legally empowered to do so in England, Wales and Northern Ireland. Nor can competent people, facing mental incapacity, nominate others to make legally binding treatment choices for them.

In Scotland, the powers of a tutor dative might fulfil such a function. The authority of a tutor dative to refuse treatment on behalf of an incompetent patient would, it is thought, depend largely on whether the refusal conformed with the patient's own wishes and whether those could be shown to be informed and applicable. No case of refusal by a tutor dative has yet been heard in Scotland, but there may be little **practical** difference when compared with the position in England, Wales and Northern Ireland.

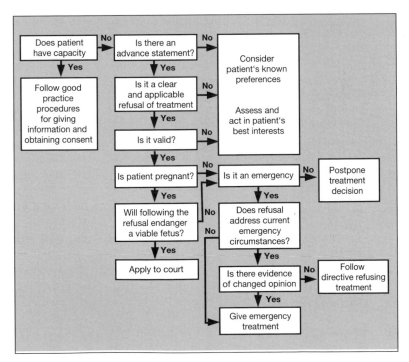

Figure 2.

10.5 If an incapacitated pregnant woman presents with an apparently valid advance directive refusing treatment, legal advice should be sought to clarify the position.

If a mentally incapacitated and clearly pregnant woman presents with an apparently valid advance directive refusing treatment, legal advice should be sought. The courts may consider the advance refusal ineffective if withholding treatment endangers an otherwise viable fetus.

10.6 One type of particularly serious condition is the persistent vegetative state (pvs) where there is no chance of recovery, but where life is dependent on artificial feeding. Diagnosis of this condition can only be made after twelve months when it is due to head injury but six months if it is due to other causes. The courts have to be consulted before treatment can be withdrawn and so any directive relating to pvs should be put before the courts before it can take effect.

10.7 If doubt exists about what the individual intends, the law supports a presumption in favour of providing clinically appropriate treatment. Carers and nurses during their working relationship with long-stay patients in residential or in-patient settings, are likely to have an understanding of the patient's feelings and opinions. Whilst these views should be taken into account they should not necessarily be determinative if in conflict with other evidence.

11 Liability of Health Professionals

11.1 Health professionals may be legally liable if they disregard the terms of an advance directive (ie refusal of treatment) if the directive is known of and applicable to the circumstances.

Health professionals following the terms of a clear advance directive (refusal of treatment) and exercising due care and attention would be very unlikely to face prosecution. The Crown

Prosecution Service in its evidence to the House of Lords has endorsed the view that if an incompetent patient had previously made an advance directive (refusal), health professionals "must abide by the terms of that previous expression of intention or wish, though special care may be necessary to ensure that any prior refusal of consent to medical treatment is still properly to be regarded as applicable in the circumstances which have subsequently occurred".[11]

This Code provides, however, that an advance refusal of the minimally essential measures necessary to keep a patient comfortable ("basic care") should not be binding (see section 5). In case of doubt, legal opinion should be sought. The Official Solicitor's office represents mentally incapacitated people's interests in legal matters and may be able to advise appropriate action, although a court ruling or declaratory judgement may be required.

Health professionals must always act with due care and attention. For example, the mistaken application of an advance refusal to a patient other than the one who made it may raise issues of negligence.

11.1.1 Applicability

If the situation is not identical to that described in the advance statement or refusal, it is still advisable to act in the general spirit of the statement, if this is clearly described. If any individuals are named in the statement for contact, they, as well as the GP may be able to clarify the patient's wishes. If there is doubt, however, as to what a patient intended, the law supports a presumption that appropriate life-prolonging measures should be given.

Health professionals must use their own professional judgement about the appropriateness of the statement. If a refusal is not applicable to the circumstances, it is not legally binding although it may still give valuable indications of the general

---

11   Report from the Select Committee on Medical Ethics, HMSO, 1994, Vol 1, p.39

treatment options the patient would prefer. If a statement requests or consents to certain options, for example, the health team will have to judge whether the treatment is medically appropriate or advisable for that patient at that time.

12 Disputes

12.1 In the event of disagreement between health professionals or between health professionals and people close to the patient, the senior clinician must consider the available evidence of the patient's wishes.

Junior medical and other staff should ensure that the senior professional managing the case is kept aware of the patient's oral wishes or written statement. There may, however, be clinical reasons for not complying with a patient's requests or preferences. A clear, applicable advance refusal will have legal force and the consultant should be informed of this. Thereafter, junior medical, nursing and other professional staff should accept the judgement of the clinician in overall charge of the patient.

12.2 In cases of doubt or disagreement about the scope or validity of an advance directive (refusal), emergency treatment should normally be given and advice sought from the courts if the matter cannot be clarified in any other way.

In the event of disagreement between health professionals or between relatives and health professionals about the patient's previously expressed wishes, opinions should be sought from relevant colleagues and others who are familiar with the patient. The point of discussion should not be to override the patient's view but to clarify its scope and seek evidence concerning its validity. Ultimately, the senior professional managing the particular episode of the patient's care should take responsibility and may need to seek advice from the courts if the matter cannot be clarified.

12.3 In any case of dispute, legal judgment will be based upon the strength of the evidence.

Disagreements may arise between a hospital doctor and a GP or between nursing and medical staff in a hospital. All staff involved in a patient's care should have an opportunity of presenting their views. From a patient's viewpoint, nurses are often the most accessible professional. Hospital or community nurses may, over a period of time, have had closer contact than others with the patient and with those close to the patient. Nurses are often adept in translating technical medical language and discussing practical aspects of outcomes of treatment and care. They may gain particular insight into whether patients were consistent and coherent in their views.

13 Conscientious Objection

13.1 Some health professionals disagree in principle with patients' rights to refuse life-prolonging treatment but may nonetheless support advance statements which express preferences.

13.2 Health professionals are entitled to have their personal moral beliefs respected and not be pressurised to act contrary to those beliefs. But the "sanctity of life" argument or other values must not be imposed upon those for whom they have or had no meaning.

13.3 Health professionals with a conscientious objection to limiting treatment at a patient's request should make their view clear when the patient initially raises the matter. In such cases the patient should be advised of the option of seeing another health professional if the patient wishes.

13.4 If a health professional is involved in the management of a case and cannot for reasons of conscience accede to a patient's request for limitation of treatment, management of that patient must be passed to a colleague.

13.5 In an emergency, if no other health professional is available there is a legal duty to comply with an appropriate and valid advance refusal.

Some doctors and nurses have moral objections to withholding life-prolonging treatment. Their views should be respected and they must not be marginalised within the health-care service. The people they care for have the right to know as far as possible how their requests or refusals will be received. Health professionals with a conscientious objection should make that clear when the patient initially raises the matter so that the patient can decide how to proceed.

Health professionals unable to limit treatment on request should step aside and pass management of that patient to a colleague. In an emergency, if delegation is impossible, the doctor or nurse must comply with a valid advance directive (treatment refusal). It is unacceptable to force treatment upon a patient.

PART V

Summary

14 Summary

14.1 Although not binding on health professionals, advance statements deserve thorough consideration and respect.

14.2 Where valid and applicable, advance directives (refusals) must be followed.

14.3 Health professionals consulted by people wishing to formulate an advance statement or directive should take all reasonable steps to provide accurate factual information about the treatment options and their implications.

14.4 Where an unknown and incapacitated patient presents for treatment some checks should be made concerning the validity of any directive refusing life-prolonging treatment. In all cases, it is vital to check that the statement or refusal presented is that of the patient being treated and has not been withdrawn.

14.5 If the situation is not identical to that described in the advance statement or refusal, treatment providers may still be guided by the general spirit of the statement if this is evident. It is advisable to contact any person nominated by the patient as well as the GP to clarify the patient's wishes. If there is doubt as to what the patient intended, the law requires the exercise of a best interests judgement.

14.6 If an incapacitated person is known to have had sustained and informed objections to all or some treatment, even though these have not been formally recorded, health professionals may not be justified in proceeding. This applies even in an emergency.

If witnessed and made at a time when the patient was competent and informed, such objections may constitute an oral advance directive. Health professionals will need to consider how much evidence is available about the patient's decisions and how convincing it seems. All members of the health care team can make a useful contribution to this process.

14.7 In the absence of any indication of the patient's wishes, there is a common law duty to give appropriate treatment to incapacitated patients when the treatment is clearly in their best interests.

Checklist for writing an advance statement

In drawing up an advance statement you must ensure, as a minimum, that the following information is included:

- Full name

- Address

- Name and address of general practitioner

- Whether advice was sought from health professionals

- Signature

- Date drafted and reviewed

- Witness signature

- A clear statement of your wishes, either general or specific

- The name, address and telephone number of your nominated person, if you have one